Understanding Child Mental Health for Parents

A Guide to Help a Child with Mental Health Crisis

By

Hallel Isaac

TABLE OF CONTENT

COPYRIGHT

CHAPTER 1

Introduction

Child mental health refers to the psychological, emotional, and social well-being of children and adolescents. It encompasses their ability to effectively cope with stress, form and maintain healthy relationships, and manage their emotions. Child mental health is crucial for their overall development and functioning, as it directly impacts their cognitive, emotional, and behavioral abilities.

Healthy child mental health enables children to:

1. Experience and express a wide range of emotions appropriately.

2. Develop age-appropriate social skills and interact positively with others.

3. Adapt to various life changes and challenges.

4. Concentrate and perform well in school or other activities.

5. Develop a positive self-image and confidence.

6. Cope with stress, anxiety, and other emotions in a healthy manner.

7. Recognize and seek help when facing mental health difficulties.

Conversely, when a child experiences challenges in their mental health, it can lead to emotional and behavioral difficulties that may interfere with their daily life and overall well-being. These challenges can manifest in various forms, such as anxiety disorders, depression, attention deficit hyperactivity disorder (ADHD), conduct disorders, and more.

Addressing child mental health is crucial for promoting healthy development, preventing long-term mental health issues, and supporting children in reaching their full potential. Early identification and appropriate interventions play a vital role in ensuring the well-being of children and improving their mental health outcomes. Mental health professionals, caregivers, educators, and communities all have a role to play in supporting child mental health and fostering a nurturing environment for children to thrive.

As of my last update in September 2021, child mental health disorders were a significant concern worldwide. Here are some key statistics and prevalence rates for child mental health disorders based on data available up to that time:

1.   Prevalence   Rates: The prevalence of child mental health disorders can vary across different countries and regions. However, on a global scale, it was estimated that about 10-20% of children and adolescents experience mental health disorders.

2. Anxiety   Disorders: Anxiety disorders were among the most

common mental health issues affecting children and adolescents. It was reported that approximately 8-10% of young people experienced some form of anxiety disorder, such as generalized anxiety disorder, social anxiety disorder, or separation anxiety disorder.

3. Depression: Depression was another significant mental health concern for children and adolescents. It was estimated that around 3-5% of young people experienced major depressive disorder (MDD) or persistent depressive disorder (dysthymia).

4. Attention-Deficit/Hyperactivity Disorder (ADHD): ADHD is a

neurodevelopmental disorder characterized by symptoms of inattention, hyperactivity, and impulsivity. It affected approximately 5-7% of children and adolescents globally.

5. Conduct Disorder: Conduct disorder is a behavioral disorder characterized by aggressive and antisocial behavior. It was

reported to affect about 2-5% of children and adolescents.

6. Autism Spectrum Disorders (ASD): ASD is a developmental disorder that affects communication, behavior, and social interaction. The prevalence of ASD was estimated to be around 1-2% in children.

7.   Eating   Disorders: Eating disorders,   such   as   anorexia nervosa and bulimia nervosa, were also prevalent among adolescents, with estimates ranging from 0.3% to 4% depending on the specific disorder and population studied.

It is essential to note that these prevalence rates are subject to change as more recent data becomes available and as awareness and understanding of child mental health disorders continue to evolve. Additionally, access to mental health services and cultural factors can influence the reporting and diagnosis of these disorders in different regions.

Child mental health disorders can have significant and long-lasting impacts on a child's overall well-being and development. Early identification, intervention, and support are crucial in addressing these issues and promoting better mental health outcomes for children and adolescents.

If you are looking for more up-to-date statistics, I recommend consulting recent reports and publications from reputable sources like the World Health Organization (WHO) or national health agencies.

CHAPTER 2

Influences of Child Mental Health

Child mental health is influenced by a complex interplay of various factors, including biological, psychological, social, and environmental elements. Understanding these factors can help identify potential risks and promote positive mental health outcomes for children. Here are some of the key factors that can influence a child's mental health:

1. Genetics and Biology: Biological factors, including genetic predisposition, can play a significant role in a child's mental health. Certain genetic factors may

increase the risk of developing mental health conditions or make a child more susceptible to specific challenges.

2. Early Childhood Experiences: Early childhood experiences, including the quality of attachment with caregivers, exposure to trauma, neglect, or adverse childhood experiences

(ACEs), can have lasting impacts on a child's mental health.

3. Family Environment: The family environment plays a crucial role in shaping a child's mental well-being. Factors such as parental support, parenting style, family communication, and the presence of conflict or violence within the family can impact a

child's emotional and psychological development.

4. Socioeconomic Status: Socioeconomic factors, such as poverty, lack of access to education, and limited resources, can contribute to stress and increase the risk of mental health issues in children.

5. Peer Relationships: Positive and supportive peer relationships can enhance a child's mental health, while negative or toxic peer interactions can lead to emotional difficulties.

6. School Environment: The school environment plays a vital role in a child's mental health. Factors like academic pressure, bullying,

teacher-student relationships, and the overall school climate can affect a child's emotional well-being.

7. Traumatic Events: Exposure to trauma, such as physical or sexual abuse, natural disasters, or witnessing violence, can have severe and long-lasting effects on a child's mental health.

8. Media and Technology: The content and amount of exposure to media and technology can impact a child's mental health. Excessive screen time, violent content, and cyberbullying can be detrimental.

9. Cultural and Societal Influences: Cultural beliefs, societal norms,

and attitudes toward mental health can influence how children perceive and express their emotions and seek help for mental health issues.

10. Access to Mental Health Services: The availability and accessibility of mental health services, including early intervention and treatment

options, can significantly impact a child's mental health outcomes.

11. Coping Skills and Resilience: A child's ability to cope with stress and adversity, as well as their level of resilience, can influence their mental health.

It is essential to recognize that these factors often interact with each other, and individual children may respond differently to various influences. Providing a nurturing, supportive, and understanding environment, along with access to appropriate mental health resources, can help promote positive mental health in children.

CHAPTER 3

Common Child Mental Health Disorders

As of my last update in September 2021, several common child mental health disorders affect children and adolescents. It's important to note that the prevalence and understanding of these disorders may evolve, so it's always best to consult the latest research and professional sources for the most up-to-date information. Here are some of the common child mental health disorders:

1. Attention-Deficit/Hyperactivity Disorder (ADHD): ADHD is

characterized by symptoms of inattention, hyperactivity, and impulsivity. Children with ADHD may struggle with staying focused, following instructions, and sitting still, which can impact their academic performance and social interactions.

2. Autism Spectrum Disorder (ASD): ASD is a neurodevelopmental disorder characterized by difficulties in social communication and repetitive patterns of behavior. Children with ASD may have challenges with social interactions, and communication skills, and may display repetitive

movements or engage in restrictive behaviors.

3. Anxiety Disorders: Anxiety disorders in children can include generalized anxiety disorder, social anxiety disorder, separation anxiety disorder, and specific phobias. Children with anxiety disorders may experience excessive worry, fear, and physical

symptoms like headaches or stomachaches related to their anxiety.

4. Depression: Childhood depression can manifest as persistent feelings of sadness, loss of interest in activities, changes in sleep or appetite, and difficulties with concentration. It's important to distinguish between normal

fluctuations in mood and more concerning signs of depression.

5. Oppositional Defiant Disorder (ODD): ODD is characterized by patterns of defiant, disobedient, and hostile behavior toward authority figures. Children with ODD may have frequent temper tantrums, be argumentative, and refuse to follow rules.

6. Conduct Disorder (CD): Conduct disorder involves more severe behavioral problems, including aggression, destruction of property, and violation of rules and rights of others. Children with CD may engage in antisocial behaviors and struggle to empathize with others' feelings.

7. Post-Traumatic Stress Disorder (PTSD): PTSD can occur in children who have experienced or witnessed traumatic events. Symptoms may include intrusive thoughts, nightmares, avoidance of reminders, and heightened arousal.

8. Obsessive-Compulsive Disorder (OCD): OCD involves intrusive,

unwanted thoughts (obsessions) and repetitive behaviors or mental acts (compulsions) performed to alleviate anxiety related to those obsessions.

9. Specific Learning Disorders: Learning disorders affect a child's ability to acquire and use specific academic skills, such as reading, writing, or mathematics. Dyslexia

is one example of a specific
learning disorder.

It's important to remember that
early detection and appropriate
intervention are crucial in
addressing child mental health
disorders. If you suspect that a
child is experiencing mental
health challenges, it's essential to
seek professional help from a

qualified mental health provider or pediatrician. They can conduct assessments, provide accurate diagnoses, and recommend suitable treatment options tailored to the child's specific needs.

CHAPTER 4

The Role of Parents, Caregivers, and Teachers in Early Detection

Parents, caregivers, and teachers play critical roles in the early detection of mental health issues in children. They are often the first line of defense in recognizing signs of distress or behavioral changes that may indicate a child is struggling with their emotional well-being. Here's how each of these individuals can contribute to early detection:

1. Parents:

   - Observation: Parents spend significant time with their children and are in a unique position to observe any changes in behavior, emotions, or social interactions.

- Communication: Open and supportive communication with their child allows parents to better understand their feelings, concerns, and struggles.

-Recognizing Changes:Parents can identify sudden shifts in

mood, withdrawal from activities, changes in sleep or appetite patterns, and expressions of excessive fear or worry.

- Seeking Professional Help: If parents notice persistent or concerning behaviors, they can take the initiative to seek professional help from a pediatrician, school counselor, or mental health specialist.

2. Caregivers (e.g., Grandparents, Extended Family, Babysitters):

- Continuity of Care: Caregivers who spend time with the child can provide valuable insights into the child's emotional and behavioral patterns, even if they are not present daily.

- Communication with Parents: Sharing observations and

concerns with the child's parents ensures that important information reaches those who can make decisions about the child's well-being.

- Supportive Role: Caregivers can provide emotional support and a safe space for the child to express their feelings and concerns.

3. Teachers:

- Daily Interaction: Teachers interact with children during a significant portion of the day, giving them a chance to observe the child's behavior in various contexts.

- Academic and Social Changes: Teachers may notice changes in academic performance, changes in participation in classroom activities, or difficulties in social interactions with peers.

- Collaboration with Parents: Teachers can communicate with parents about any observed changes or concerns, working together to support the child's well-being.

- School-Based Interventions: Teachers can initiate or participate in school-based interventions, such as counseling or referral to the school's support team, to address the child's needs.

In the context of early detection, parents, caregivers, and teachers need to maintain open lines of communication. Sharing observations and concerns and working collaboratively can lead to a more comprehensive understanding of the child's overall well-being.

Additionally, providing resources and information to parents, caregivers, and teachers about common signs of mental health issues in children can empower them to recognize potential red flags. These may include sudden changes in behavior, persistent sadness, excessive worries or fears, difficulty concentrating, social withdrawal, changes in sleep or eating habits, or expressions of hopelessness.

Early detection allows for timely intervention and support, which can significantly improve the child's mental health outcomes. If any concerns arise, seeking guidance from a qualified mental health professional is essential to assess the child's needs and provide appropriate care.

Challenges in recognizing mental health problems in children

Recognizing mental health problems in children can be challenging due to various factors. Some of the key challenges include:

1. Limited Awareness and Knowledge: Many parents,

caregivers, and even teachers may lack awareness and knowledge about the signs and symptoms of mental health issues in children. They may mistake certain behaviors as typical developmental phases or misunderstand the seriousness of the child's distress.

2. Communication Barriers: Young children, especially those who haven't fully developed their language skills, may struggle to express their emotions or describe what they are going through. They may not have the words to articulate their feelings, making it harder for adults to understand their inner struggles.

3. Developmental Variability: Children's mental health symptoms can manifest differently based on their age, developmental stage, and individual differences. This variability can make it challenging to identify consistent patterns of concern.

4. Stigma and Fear of Labeling: Stigma surrounding mental health issues can deter parents and caregivers from acknowledging potential problems in their children. They may fear the judgment or labeling associated with seeking help for mental health concerns.

5.   Normalizing   Problematic Behaviors: Certain   behavioral issues   or   emotional   struggles might   be   normalized   or overlooked as "just a phase" or typical childhood behavior. As a result, underlying mental health problems may go unrecognized.

6. Co-Occurrence of Disorders: Children with mental health issues

may experience multiple conditions simultaneously, making it harder to identify specific problems. For example, anxiety and depression might coexist, making the diagnostic process more complex.

7. Masking in Different Settings: A child's mental health problems might be more evident in one

setting (e.g., home) while remaining hidden in another (e.g., school). This can lead to inconsistent observations, making it challenging to pinpoint the root cause of the child's difficulties.

8. Overlapping Symptoms with Physical Health Issues: Some mental health symptoms, such as headaches, stomachaches, or

changes in sleep patterns, can be mistaken for physical health problems, delaying the recognition of the underlying mental health concern.

9. Resistance to Seeking Help: Children, especially adolescents, may resist seeking help for mental health issues due to fear, denial, or

a desire to appear "normal" to their peers.

10. Cultural and Societal Factors: Cultural beliefs and societal norms can influence how mental health problems are perceived and addressed. In some cultures, mental health issues may be stigmatized, leading to hesitancy in seeking professional support.

To overcome these challenges, it's essential to increase mental health literacy among parents, caregivers, and teachers. Educating them about common signs of mental health issues in children and encouraging open and supportive communication can help facilitate early detection and intervention.

Additionally, involving mental health professionals in the assessment process can provide a more comprehensive understanding of the child's well-being and lead to appropriate support and treatment.

CHAPTER 5

Impact of Child Mental Health on Development

Child mental health has a significant impact on various aspects of a child's development. The early years of a child's life are crucial for their emotional, social, cognitive, and physical development. When mental health issues arise during this period, they can have long-lasting effects that can extend into adulthood. Here are some key areas where child mental health can influence development:

1. Emotional Development: Mental health plays a vital role in emotional regulation and

resilience. Children with good mental health are more likely to develop a stable emotional foundation, enabling them to cope with stress, form positive relationships, and adapt to new situations. Conversely, children experiencing mental health challenges may struggle with emotional regulation, leading to frequent mood swings, anxiety, or depression.

2. Cognitive Development: Child mental health impacts cognitive abilities, including attention, memory, problem-solving, and academic performance. Children facing mental health issues might find it difficult to concentrate,

leading to challenges in learning and educational achievement.

3. Social Development: Interacting with others is a critical aspect of child development. Healthy mental health facilitates positive social interactions, empathy, and communication skills. Conversely, children with mental health difficulties may struggle with

forming and maintaining relationships, leading to feelings of isolation or withdrawal from social activities.

4. Physical Health: Mental health and physical health are interconnected. Chronic stress and mental health issues can contribute to physical health problems and weaken the immune

system. Additionally, unhealthy coping mechanisms such as substance abuse might arise as a result of untreated mental health issues, further affecting physical well-being.

5. Parent-Child Relationships: The mental health of caregivers and parents can also impact child development. If parents are

experiencing mental health challenges, it can affect their ability to provide consistent and supportive caregiving, which is crucial for a child's emotional and psychological growth.

6. Long-term Outcomes: Early mental health issues that go untreated can have lasting effects on an individual's life trajectory.

Children who experience mental health problems are at a higher risk of academic underachievement, substance abuse, delinquency, and difficulties in forming stable relationships in adulthood.

7. Resilience: Positive mental health is linked to resilience, the ability to bounce back from challenges and adversities. Children with good mental health are more likely to develop coping skills and resilience, which helps them navigate life's ups and downs more effectively.

Addressing child mental health issues early is crucial to supporting healthy development. Early intervention, therapy, and support services can be effective in mitigating the negative impact of mental health challenges and promoting positive growth and well-being in children. Parents, caregivers, educators, and healthcare professionals need to be vigilant for signs of mental health difficulties and seek appropriate help when needed.

CHAPTER 6

Treatment and Interventions for Child Mental Health

Treatment and interventions for a child's mental health can vary based on the specific mental health condition or issue the child is facing. It's essential to recognize that each child is unique, and the appropriate approach will depend on factors such as the child's age, the severity of the condition, and their individual needs. Here are some common treatment and intervention options for child mental health:

1. Psychotherapy (Talk Therapy): This involves working with a

trained therapist or counselor who specializes in child mental health. Different types of therapy may be used, such as cognitive-behavioral therapy (CBT), play therapy (for younger children), family therapy, or art therapy. Psychotherapy can help children explore their feelings, thoughts, and behaviors and develop coping strategies.

2. Medication: In some cases, a child's mental health condition may require medication to manage symptoms effectively. This is typically determined by a child psychiatrist or pediatrician with expertise in child mental health. Medication is often used in conjunction with other therapies for optimal results.

3. Behavioral Interventions: These interventions aim to modify and shape a child's behavior through positive reinforcement, rewards, and consequences. They can help address behavioral issues, attention problems, and certain mood disorders.

4. Parent Training and Support: Involving parents in the treatment process is crucial for the child's well-being. Parent training programs can teach parents effective strategies for managing their child's behavior, communication skills, and emotional support.

5. School-based Interventions: Teachers and school staff play an essential role in supporting a child's mental health. School-based interventions can include classroom accommodations, counseling services within the school setting, and collaboration with parents to create a supportive environment for the child.

6. Group Therapy: Group therapy can provide children with a safe space to connect with peers who may be experiencing similar challenges. It can help improve social skills, build self-esteem, and reduce feelings of isolation.

7. Mindfulness and Relaxation Techniques: Teaching children

mindfulness and relaxation techniques can help them manage stress, anxiety, and emotional difficulties. Techniques like deep breathing, meditation, and yoga can be beneficial.

8. Supportive Services: In some cases, additional support services may be necessary, such as occupational therapy, speech

therapy, or specialized programs for specific conditions like autism spectrum disorder.

9. Early Intervention Programs: Early identification and intervention are essential for promoting positive mental health outcomes in children. Early intervention programs aim to identify and address

developmental or behavioral concerns as early as possible.

10. Community Resources and Support: Connecting families to community resources and support networks can be valuable in sustaining the child's progress and providing ongoing assistance.

It's important to note that seeking professional help is vital for accurate assessment and to develop a personalized treatment plan tailored to the child's needs.

If you are concerned about a child's mental health, consider reaching out to a qualified mental health professional or your pediatrician for guidance and support.

CHAPTER 7

Challenges and Barriers to Accessing

Mental Health Care

Accessing mental health care can be challenging for various reasons, and these challenges can act as significant barriers to individuals seeking the help they need. Some of the common challenges and barriers include:

1. Stigma and Discrimination: The stigma surrounding mental health issues can lead to shame and fear of judgment, causing individuals to avoid seeking help.

Stigmatizing attitudes in society can prevent people from openly discussing their struggles and deter them from accessing mental health care.

2. Limited Mental Health Services: In many regions, there is a shortage of mental health professionals, especially in rural or underserved areas. This lack of resources can result in long

waiting lists and limited access to specialized care.

3. Cost and Insurance Coverage: Mental health services can be expensive, and not everyone has adequate insurance coverage for mental health care. High out-of-pocket costs may prevent individuals from seeking treatment or accessing ongoing therapy.

4. Lack of Awareness and Education: Some people may not recognize the signs of mental health issues or may not understand that mental health care is essential for overall well-being. Lack of awareness and education can delay help-seeking behavior.

5. Language and Cultural Barriers: Language differences and cultural beliefs can create barriers to accessing mental health care. People from diverse backgrounds may feel uncomfortable or misunderstood when seeking help.

6. Transportation and Accessibility: Limited access to transportation, particularly in

rural or low-income areas, can make it difficult for individuals to reach mental health facilities or providers.

7. Fear of Hospitalization or Involuntary Treatment: Some individuals may be hesitant to seek help due to a fear of hospitalization or involuntary

treatment, which they perceive as losing control over their lives.

8. Long Wait Times: Even in areas with mental health services available, long wait times for appointments can be discouraging and harmful, particularly for those in crisis.

9. Mental Health Literacy: People may lack knowledge about available treatment options, leading them to avoid seeking care or relying on ineffective or harmful methods.

10. Lack of Integration with Primary Care: Mental health care is sometimes not well integrated into primary care settings, making

it less accessible and resulting in missed opportunities for early intervention.

11. Child and Adolescent Mental Health Services: Access to mental health care for children and adolescents can be particularly challenging due to a shortage of child mental health specialists and appropriate resources.

Addressing these challenges requires a multi-faceted approach, including reducing stigma through education and awareness campaigns, increasing funding and resources for mental health services, improving insurance coverage for mental health care, expanding telehealth options to reach underserved areas, and integrating mental health care into primary care settings. Additionally, culturally sensitive and inclusive practices can help bridge gaps in access for individuals from diverse backgrounds.

CHAPTER 8

Promoting Child Mental Health

Promoting child mental health is essential for fostering the well-being and healthy development of children. Here are some strategies and practices that can help promote child mental health:

1. Early Intervention: Identify and address mental health concerns as early as possible. Early intervention can prevent issues from escalating and provide support when children need it most.

2. Create Safe and Nurturing Environments: Ensure that

children have safe and supportive environments at home, school, and in the community. Positive relationships with parents, caregivers, teachers, and peers contribute to a child's emotional well-being.

3. Promote Positive Parenting: Provide parents and caregivers with resources and support to

enhance their parenting skills. Positive parenting practices, such as emotional responsiveness and setting appropriate boundaries, can positively influence a child's mental health.

4. Emotional Expression and Communication: Encourage children to express their emotions openly and provide them with the

tools to communicate their feelings effectively. This can help reduce emotional bottling and enhance emotional intelligence.

5. Promote Healthy Lifestyle Habits: Encourage regular physical activity, balanced nutrition, and sufficient sleep. A healthy lifestyle supports mental and emotional well-being.

6. Reduce Stressors: Minimize stressors in children's lives and teach them effective coping strategies to manage stress. Excessive stress can impact a child's mental health negatively.

7. Develop Social Skills: Help children develop social skills and build strong peer relationships.

Social competence is essential for emotional resilience and overall mental well-being.

8. Foster a Positive School Environment: Schools play a significant role in promoting child mental health. Implement anti-bullying programs, provide support services, and create a

positive and inclusive school climate.

9. Education and Awareness: Increase mental health literacy among parents, teachers, and the community. Promote awareness of child mental health issues and reduce stigma through education and open discussions.

10. Screening and Assessment: Regularly screen and assess children's mental health to identify potential concerns early on. This allows for timely intervention and support.

11. Access to Mental Health Services: Improve access to affordable and quality mental health services for children. This

includes increasing the number of child mental health professionals and integrating mental health care into primary care settings and schools.

12. Promote Play and Creativity: Encourage children to engage in imaginative play and creative activities. Play can be therapeutic

and beneficial for a child's emotional well-being.

13. Family Involvement: Involve families in the child's mental health care and treatment. Collaboration between parents, caregivers, and mental health professionals is crucial for successful outcomes.

14. Limit Screen Time: Set appropriate limits on screen time and encourage more interactive and face-to-face activities. Excessive screen time can impact children's mental health and social development.

Promoting child mental health requires a comprehensive and collaborative effort involving families, educators, healthcare providers, policymakers, and the community. By prioritizing the mental well-being of children, we can help them grow into emotionally resilient and mentally healthy individuals.

CHAPTER 9

The Way Out

Addressing child mental health issues requires a collective and concerted effort from individuals, communities, policymakers, and organizations. Here's a call to action to promote the mental well-being of children:

1. Raise Awareness: Start by raising awareness about the importance of child mental health. Spread information about the prevalence of mental health issues in children and the potential long-term impact on their lives.

2. Break the Stigma: Challenge the stigma surrounding mental health by promoting open discussions

and understanding. Encourage empathy and compassion for children and families dealing with mental health challenges.

3. Invest in Mental Health Services: Advocate for increased funding and resources to improve access to mental health services for children. This includes expanding the number of child

mental health professionals and facilities.

4. Integrate Mental Health into Education: Work with schools to integrate mental health education and support into the curriculum. Train teachers and staff to recognize signs of distress and provide appropriate referrals.

5. Promote Parent and Caregiver Education: Provide workshops and resources to parents and caregivers to help them recognize signs of mental health issues in children and understand how to support their child's well-being.

6. Screening and Early Intervention: Implement routine mental health screening in schools

and healthcare settings to identify potential issues early. Early intervention can prevent problems from worsening and promote better outcomes.

7. Supportive Environments: Create safe and supportive environments for children at home, school, and in the community. Positive relationships

and nurturing surroundings are vital for a child's emotional development.

8. Prioritize School-Based Mental Health Programs: Support the implementation of comprehensive school-based mental health programs, including counseling services, support groups, and anti-bullying initiatives.

9. Telehealth and Digital Mental Health Solutions: Advocate for the expansion of telehealth services and digital mental health platforms to increase access to care, particularly in underserved areas.

10. Involve the Community: Engage community organizations,

religious institutions, and local leaders to collaborate on mental health initiatives. Community support can foster resilience in children and families.

11. Support Research and Data Collection: Encourage research on child mental health issues to better understand the challenges

and develop evidence-based interventions.

12. Advocate for Policy Changes: Work with policymakers to advocate for policies that prioritize child mental health, including insurance coverage for mental health services and increased funding for mental health programs.

13.   Promote   Parent-Child Communication: Encourage open and supportive communication between parents and children about emotions and mental health. Teach parents to be active listeners and create a safe space for children to express their feelings.

14. Address Trauma and Adverse Childhood Experiences (ACEs): Advocate for trauma-informed practices and programs that address adverse childhood experiences, as these can have a significant impact on a child's mental health.

15. Celebrate Success Stories: Highlight success stories of

children who have overcome mental health challenges and thrived with the right support. **Positive examples can inspire hope and reduce stigma.**

Remember that addressing child mental health issues is an ongoing process that requires collaboration and commitment from all stakeholders. By working together, we can create a nurturing and supportive environment that promotes the well-being of every child and ensures they have the opportunity to reach their full potential.

emotional and psychological development.

4.   Socioeconomic Status: Socioeconomic factors, such as

poverty, lack of access to education, and limited resources, can contribute to stress and increase the risk of mental health issues in children.

5. Peer Relationships: Positive and supportive peer relationships can enhance a child's mental health, while negative or toxic peer

interactions can lead to emotional difficulties.

6. School Environment: The school environment plays a vital role in a child's mental health. Factors like academic pressure, bullying, teacher-student relationships, and the overall school climate can affect a child's emotional well-being.

7. Traumatic Events: Exposure to trauma, such as physical or sexual abuse, natural disasters, or witnessing violence, can have severe and long-lasting effects on a child's mental health.

8. Media and Technology: The content and amount of exposure to media and technology can

impact a child's mental health. Excessive screen time, violent content, and cyberbullying can be detrimental.

9. Cultural and Societal Influences: Cultural beliefs, societal norms, and attitudes toward mental health can influence how children perceive and express their

emotions and seek help for mental health issues.

10. Access to Mental Health Services: The availability and accessibility of mental health services, including early intervention and treatment options, can significantly impact a child's mental health outcomes.

11. Coping Skills and Resilience: A child's ability to cope with stress and adversity, as well as their level of resilience, can influence their mental health.

It is essential to recognize that these factors often interact with each other, and individual children may respond differently to various influences. Providing a nurturing, supportive, and understanding environment, along with access to appropriate mental health resources, can help promote positive mental health in children.